Table of Contents

Introduction

Diabetes is a condition that impairs the body's ability to process blood glucose, otherwise known as blood sugar.

In the United States, the estimated number of people over 18 years of age with diagnosed and undiagnosed diabetes is 30.2 million. The figure represents between 27.9 and 32.7 percent of the population.

Without ongoing, careful management, diabetes can lead to a buildup of sugars in the blood, which can increase the risk of dangerous complications, including stroke and heart disease.

Different kinds of diabetes can occur, and managing the condition depends on the type. Not all forms of diabetes stem from a person being overweight or leading an inactive lifestyle. In fact, some are present from childhood.

Diabetes types

Diabetes mellitus, commonly known as diabetes, is a metabolic disease that causes high blood sugar. The hormone insulin moves sugar from the blood into your cells to be stored or used for energy. With diabetes, your body either doesn't make enough insulin or can't effectively use the insulin it does make.

Untreated high blood sugar from diabetes can damage your nerves, eyes, kidneys, and other organs.

There are a few different types of diabetes:

• Type 1 diabetes is an autoimmune disease. The immune system attacks and destroys cells in the pancreas, where insulin is made. It's unclear what causes this attack. About 10 percent of people with diabetes have this type.

• Type 2 diabetes occurs when your body becomes resistant to insulin, and sugar builds up in your blood.

• Prediabetes occurs when your blood sugar is higher than normal, but it's not high enough for a diagnosis of type 2 diabetes.

• Gestational diabetes is high blood sugar during pregnancy. Insulin-blocking hormones produced by the placenta cause this type of diabetes.

A rare condition called diabetes insipidus is not related to diabetes mellitus, although it has a similar name. It's a different condition in which your kidneys remove too much fluid from your body.

Each type of diabetes has unique symptoms, causes, and treatments.

Prediabetes

Doctors refer to some people as having prediabetes or borderline diabetes when blood sugar is usually in the range of 100 to 125 milligrams per deciliter (mg/dL).

Normal blood sugar levels sit between 70 and 99 mg/dL, whereas a person with diabetes will have a fasting blood sugar higher than 126 mg/dL.

The prediabetes level means that blood glucose is higher than usual but not so high as to constitute diabetes.

People with prediabetes are, however, at risk of developing type 2 diabetes, although they do not usually experience the symptoms of full diabetes.

The risk factors for prediabetes and type 2 diabetes are similar. They include:

• being overweight

• a family history of diabetes

• having a high-density lipoprotein (HDL) cholesterol level lower than 40 mg/dL or 50 mg/dL

• a history of high blood pressure

• having gestational diabetes or giving birth to a child with a birth weight of more than 9 pounds

• a history of polycystic ovary syndrome (PCOS)

• being of African-American, Native American, Latin American, or Asian-Pacific Islander descent

• being more than 45 years of age

• having a sedentary lifestyle

If a doctor identifies that a person has prediabetes, they will recommend that the individual makes healthful changes that can ideally stop the progression to type 2 diabetes. Losing weight and having a more healthful diet can often help prevent the disease.

How insulin problems develop

Doctors do not know the exact causes of type I diabetes. Type 2 diabetes, also known as insulin resistance, has clearer causes.

Insulin allows the glucose from a person's food to access the cells in their body to supply energy. Insulin resistance is usually a result of the following cycle:

1. A person has genes or an environment that make it more likely that they are unable to make enough insulin to cover how much glucose they eat.

2. The body tries to make extra insulin to process the excess blood glucose.

3. The pancreas cannot keep up with the increased demands, and the excess blood sugar starts to circulate in the blood, causing damage.

4. Over time, insulin becomes less effective at introducing glucose to cells, and blood sugar levels continue to rise.

Symptoms of diabetes

Diabetes symptoms are caused by rising blood sugar.

General symptoms

The general symptoms of diabetes include:

• increased hunger

• increased thirst

• weight loss

• frequent urination

• blurry vision

• extreme fatigue

• sores that don't heal

Symptoms in men

In addition to the general symptoms of diabetes, men with diabetes may have a decreased sex drive, erectile dysfunction (ED), and poor muscle strength.

Symptoms in women

Women with diabetes can also have symptoms such as urinary tract infections, yeast infections, and dry, itchy skin.

Type 1 diabetes

Symptoms of type 1 diabetes can include:

• extreme hunger

• increased thirst

• unintentional weight loss

- frequent urination

- blurry vision

- tiredness

It may also result in mood changes.

Type 2 diabetes

Symptoms of type 2 diabetes can include:

- increased hunger

- increased thirst

- increased urination

- blurry vision

- tiredness

- sores that are slow to heal

It may also cause recurring infections. This is because elevated glucose levels make it harder for the body to heal.

Gestational diabetes

Most women with gestational diabetes don't have any symptoms. The condition is often detected during a routine blood sugar test or oral glucose tolerance test that is usually performed between the 24th and 28th weeks of gestation.

In rare cases, a woman with gestational diabetes will also experience increased thirst or urination.

The bottom line

Diabetes symptoms can be so mild that they're hard to spot at first. Learn which signs should prompt a trip to the doctor.

Causes of diabetes

Different causes are associated with each type of diabetes.

Type 1 diabetes

Doctors don't know exactly what causes type 1 diabetes. For some reason, the immune system mistakenly attacks and destroys insulin-producing beta cells in the pancreas.

Genes may play a role in some people. It's also possible that a virus sets off the immune system attack.

Type 2 diabetes

Type 2 diabetes stems from a combination of genetics and lifestyle factors. Being overweight or obese increases your risk too. Carrying extra weight, especially in your belly, makes your cells more resistant to the effects of insulin on your blood sugar.

This condition runs in families. Family members share genes that make them more likely to get type 2 diabetes and to be overweight.

Gestational diabetes

Gestational diabetes is the result of hormonal changes during pregnancy. The placenta produces hormones that make a pregnant woman's cells less sensitive to the effects of insulin. This can cause high blood sugar during pregnancy.

Women who are overweight when they get pregnant or who gain too much weight during their pregnancy are more likely to get gestational diabetes.

The bottom line

Both genes and environmental factors play a role in triggering diabetes. Get more information here on the causes of diabetes.

Diabetes risk factors

Certain factors increase your risk for diabetes.

Type 1 diabetes

You're more likely to get type 1 diabetes if you're a child or teenager, you have a parent or sibling with the condition, or you carry certain genes that are linked to the disease.

Type 2 diabetes

Your risk for type 2 diabetes increases if you:

- are overweight

- are age 45 or older

- have a parent or sibling with the condition

- aren't physically active

- have had gestational diabetes

• have prediabetes

• have high blood pressure, high cholesterol, or high triglycerides

• have African American, Hispanic or Latino American, Alaska Native, Pacific Islander, American Indian, or Asian American ancestry

Gestational diabetes

Your risk for gestational diabetes increases if you:

• are overweight

• are over age 25

• had gestational diabetes during a past pregnancy

• have given birth to a baby weighing more than 9 pounds

• have a family history of type 2 diabetes

• have polycystic ovary syndrome (PCOS)

The bottom line

Your family, environment, and preexisting medical conditions can all affect your odds of developing diabetes. Find out which risks you can control and which ones you can't.

Diabetes complications

High blood sugar damages organs and tissues throughout your body. The higher your blood sugar is and the longer you live with it, the greater your risk for complications.

Complications associated with diabetes include:

- heart disease, heart attack, and stroke

- neuropathy

- nephropathy

- retinopathy and vision loss

- hearing loss

- foot damage such as infections and sores that don't heal

- skin conditions such as bacterial and fungal infections

- depression

- dementia

Gestational diabetes

Uncontrolled gestational diabetes can lead to problems that affect both the mother and baby. Complications affecting the baby can include:

- premature birth

- higher-than-normal weight at birth

- increased risk for type 2 diabetes later in life

- low blood sugar

- jaundice

- stillbirth

The mother can develop complications such as high blood pressure (preeclampsia) or type 2 diabetes. She may also require cesarean delivery, commonly referred to as a C-section.

The mother's risk of gestational diabetes in future pregnancies also increases.

The bottom line

Diabetes can lead to serious medical complications, but you can manage the condition with medications and lifestyle changes. Avoid the most common diabetes complications with these helpful tips.

Treatment of diabetes

Doctors treat diabetes with a few different medications. Some of these drugs are taken by mouth, while others are available as injections.

Type 1 diabetes

Insulin is the main treatment for type 1 diabetes. It replaces the hormone your body isn't able to produce.

There are four types of insulin that are most commonly used. They're differentiated by how quickly they start to work, and how long their effects last:

• Rapid-acting insulin starts to work within 15 minutes and its effects last for 3 to 4 hours.

• Short-acting insulin starts to work within 30 minutes and lasts 6 to 8 hours.

• Intermediate-acting insulin starts to work within 1 to 2 hours and lasts 12 to 18 hours.

• Long-acting insulin starts to work a few hours after injection and lasts 24 hours or longer.

Type 2 diabetes

Diet and exercise can help some people manage type 2 diabetes. If lifestyle changes aren't enough to lower your blood sugar, you'll need to take medication.

These drugs lower your blood sugar in a variety of ways:

Types of drug How they work Example(s)

Alpha-glucosidase inhibitors

Slow your body's breakdown of sugars and starchy foods Acarbose (Precose) and miglitol (Glyset)

Biguanides Reduce the amount of glucose your liver makes Metformin (Glucophage)

DPP-4 inhibitors Improve your blood sugar without making it drop too low Linagliptin (Tradjenta), saxagliptin (Onglyza), and sitagliptin (Januvia)

Glucagon-like peptides Change the way your body produces insulin Dulaglutide (Trulicity), exenatide (Byetta), and liraglutide (Victoza)

Meglitinides Stimulate your pancreas to release more insulin Nateglinide (Starlix) and repaglinide (Prandin)

SGLT2 inhibitors Release more glucose into the urine Canagliflozin (Invokana) and dapagliflozin (Farxiga)

Sulfonylureas Stimulate your pancreas to release more insulin Glyburide (DiaBeta, Glynase), glipizide (Glucotrol), and glimepiride (Amaryl)

Thiazolidinediones Help insulin work better Pioglitazone (Actos) and rosiglitazone (Avandia)

You may need to take more than one of these drugs. Some people with type 2 diabetes also take insulin.

Gestational diabetes

You'll need to monitor your blood sugar level several times a day during pregnancy. If it's high, dietary changes and exercise may or may not be enough to bring it down.

According to the Mayo Clinic, about 10 to 20 percent of women with gestational diabetes will need insulin to lower their blood sugar. Insulin is safe for the growing baby.

The bottom line

The drug or combination of drugs that your doctor prescribes will depend on the type of diabetes you have — and its cause. Check out this list of the various medications that are available to treat diabetes.

Diabetes and diet

Healthy eating is a central part of managing diabetes. In some cases, changing your diet may be enough to control the disease.

Type 1 diabetes

Your blood sugar level rises or falls based on the types of foods you eat. Starchy or sugary foods make blood sugar levels rise rapidly. Protein and fat cause more gradual increases.

Your medical team may recommend that you limit the amount of carbohydrates you eat each day. You'll also need to balance your carb intake with your insulin doses.

Work with a dietitian who can help you design a diabetes meal plan. Getting the right balance of protein, fat, and carbs can help you control your blood sugar. Check out this guide to starting a type 1 diabetes diet.

Type 2 diabetes

Eating the right types of foods can both control your blood sugar and help you lose any excess weight.

Carb counting is an important part of eating for type 2 diabetes. A dietitian can help you figure out how many grams of carbohydrates to eat at each meal.

In order to keep your blood sugar levels steady, try to eat small meals throughout the day. Emphasize healthy foods such as:

• fruits

• vegetables

• whole grains

• lean protein such as poultry and fish

• healthy fats such as olive oil and nuts

Certain other foods can undermine efforts to keep your blood sugar in control. Discover the foods you should avoid if you have diabetes.

Gestational diabetes

Eating a well-balanced diet is important for both you and your baby during these nine months. Making the right food choices can also help you avoid diabetes medications.

Watch your portion sizes, and limit sugary or salty foods. Although you need some sugar to feed your growing baby, you should avoid eating too much.

Consider making an eating plan with the help of a dietitian or nutritionist. They'll ensure that your diet has the right mix of macronutrients. Go here for other do's and don'ts for healthy eating with gestational diabetes.

Diabetes diagnosis

Anyone who has symptoms of diabetes or is at risk for the disease should be tested. Women are routinely tested for gestational diabetes during their second or third trimesters of pregnancy.

Doctors use these blood tests to diagnose prediabetes and diabetes:

• The fasting plasma glucose (FPG) test measures your blood sugar after you've fasted for 8 hours.

• The A1C test provides a snapshot of your blood sugar levels over the previous 3 months.

To diagnose gestational diabetes, your doctor will test your blood sugar levels between the 24th and 28th weeks of your pregnancy.

• During the glucose challenge test, your blood sugar is checked an hour after you drink a sugary liquid.

• During the 3 hour glucose tolerance test, your blood sugar is checked after you fast overnight and then drink a sugary liquid.

The earlier you get diagnosed with diabetes, the sooner you can start treatment. Find out whether you should get tested, and get more information on tests your doctor might perform.

Diabetes prevention

Type 1 diabetes isn't preventable because it's caused by a problem with the immune system. Some causes of type 2 diabetes, such as your genes or age, aren't under your control either.

Yet many other diabetes risk factors are controllable. Most diabetes prevention strategies involve making simple adjustments to your diet and fitness routine.

If you've been diagnosed with prediabetes, here are a few things you can do to delay or prevent type 2 diabetes:

• Get at least 150 minutes per week of aerobic exercise, such as walking or cycling.

• Cut saturated and trans fats, along with refined carbohydrates, out of your diet.

• Eat more fruits, vegetables, and whole grains.

• Eat smaller portions.

• Try to lose 7 percentTrusted Source of your body weight if you're overweight or obese.

These aren't the only ways to prevent diabetes. Discover more strategies that may help you avoid this chronic disease.

Diabetes in pregnancy

Women who've never had diabetes can suddenly develop gestational diabetes in pregnancy. Hormones produced by the placenta can make your body more resistant to the effects of insulin.

Some women who had diabetes before they conceived carry it with them into pregnancy. This is called pre-gestational diabetes.

Gestational diabetes should go away after you deliver, but it does significantly increase your risk for getting diabetes later.

About half of women with gestational diabetes will develop type 2 diabetes within 5 to 10 years of delivery, according to the International Diabetes Federation (IDF).

Having diabetes during your pregnancy can also lead to complications for your newborn, such as jaundice or breathing problems.

If you're diagnosed with pre-gestational or gestational diabetes, you'll need special monitoring to prevent complications. Find out more about the effect of diabetes on pregnancy.

Diabetes in children

Children can get both type 1 and type 2 diabetes. Controlling blood sugar is especially important in young people, because the disease can damage important organs such as the heart and kidneys.

Type 1 diabetes

The autoimmune form of diabetes often starts in childhood. One of the main symptoms is increased urination. Kids with type 1 diabetes may start wetting the bed after they've been toilet trained.

Extreme thirst, fatigue, and hunger are also signs of the condition. It's important that children with type 1 diabetes get treated right away. The disease can cause high blood sugar and dehydration, which can be medical emergencies.

Type 2 diabetes

Type 1 diabetes used to be called "juvenile diabetes" because type 2 was so rare in children. Now that more children are overweight or obese, type 2 diabetes is becoming more common in this age group.

About 40 percent of children with type 2 diabetes don't have symptoms, according to the Mayo Clinic. The disease is often diagnosed during a physical exam.

Untreated type 2 diabetes can cause lifelong complications, including heart disease, kidney disease, and blindness. Healthy eating and exercise can help your child manage their blood sugar and prevent these problems.

Type 2 diabetes is more prevalent than ever in young people.

Can CBD Oil Be Used to Treat or Prevent Diabetes? What the Research Says

- Potential effectiveness

- Unproven areas

- How to take

- Side effects

- Talk to a doctor

- Legality

- Takeaway

The use of CBD oil as a treatment for diabetes — as well as epilepsy, anxiety, and a wide range of other health conditions — is showing promise, though research is still limited.

CBD is short for cannabidiol, a compound found in the Cannabis sativa plant. The other major compound is tetrahydrocannabinol (THC), the ingredient that produces a "high." CBD has no such psychoactive properties.

Among the ongoing areas of research are whether CBD oil may help treat or even lower the risk of developing both type 1 and type 2 diabetes.

Animal and human studies have looked at CBD's effects on levels of insulin, blood glucose (sugar), and inflammation, as well as complications of diabetes, such as the pain associated with diabetic neuropathy.

Read on to learn the results of these studies and how you might use CBD to potentially help prevent diabetes or alleviate some of its symptoms.

CBD oil may improve diabetes prevention, inflammation, and pain

CBD associated with improvements CBD not yet shown to be effective

diabetes prevention HDL cholesterol levels

inflammation blood glucose levels

pain

Type 1 and type 2 diabetes differ in their origin and treatment, but they present the same problem: too much glucose circulating in the blood.

Our bodies use the hormone insulin to help regulate blood glucose levels. When you eat, the pancreas produces insulin, which acts as a key, unlocking certain cells to allow glucose from the foods and beverages you consume to enter the cells to be used for energy later.

About 5 percent of people with diabetes have type 1, which occurs when the body produces little or no insulin. This means glucose remains in the bloodstream, injuring blood vessels and depriving cells of fuel.

The vast majority of diabetes cases are type 2 diabetes, which develops when cells no longer respond to insulin. That's called insulin resistance, and the result is also too much circulating glucose. Insulin resistance also boosts inflammation levels in the body.

Research findings are mixed when it comes to whether CBD oil can have a positive effect on diabetes symptoms and complications. CBD has been associated with improvements in the following:

Diabetes prevention

There have been no clinical trials to test whether CBD oil consumption can actual lower the risk of developing diabetes in humans.

However, a study in the journal Autoimmunity found that no obese diabetic (NOD) mice had a substantially lower risk of developing diabetes if treated with CBD.

Inflammation

CBD has been studied as an anti-inflammatory treatment for several years.

In a study specifically looking at inflammation triggered by high glucose levels, researchers found that CBD had positive effects on several markers of inflammation.

This study suggests that CBD may be helpful in offsetting the damage diabetes can inflict on the walls of blood vessels.

Pain

A 2017 study of rats in the journal Pain found that CBD helped reduce inflammation and nerve pain associated with osteoarthritis.

Another study, published in the Journal of Experimental Medicine, showed CBD was effective in suppressing chronic inflammatory and neuropathic pain in rodents.

CBD's effectiveness not yet proven in these areas

There's no evidence yet (although research is ongoing) that CBD oil is effective at improving HDL cholesterol levels or managing blood glucose.

HDL cholesterol

In a small 2016 study in the journal Diabetes Care, researchers found CBD oil use had little impact on HDL ("good") cholesterol levels and several other markers, such as insulin sensitivity and appetite, on people with type 2 diabetes.

Blood glucose

When it comes to potential diabetes treatments, the biggest concern is how it may help manage blood glucose levels.

At this point, there are no significant studies confirming CBD oil as a means of reducing high levels of blood sugar.

Other medications, such as metformin — together with a healthy diet and exercise — should be the main focus of your diabetes treatment and management. And if you need insulin, continue taking it as prescribed by your doctor.

How do you take CBD oil?

CBD oil is produced by extracting CBD from the cannabis plant and diluting it with a carrier oil, such as coconut or hemp seed oil.

The concentration of CBD oil varies from product to product, and there is little regulation of CBD products by the Food and Drug Administration (FDA).

Forms of CBD

Forms of CBD that you can use to potentially relieve symptoms of diabetes include:

• Vaping. Inhaling vaporized CBD oil (with the use of vaping pens or e-cigarettes) is the fastest way to experience effects. Compounds are absorbed directly from the lungs into the bloodstream.

• Oils and tinctures. Oils placed (via eye dropper) under the tongue absorb quickly into the bloodstream. Drops can also be added to foods or beverages.

• Edibles. These gummy-like candies or chocolates are good options for those who have trouble swallowing pills. Time from ingestion to effect can take a while.

• Pills and capsules. CBD pills and capsules contain a version of an oil or tincture. The time from ingestion to effect can take a while.

• Skin creams and lotions. Topical CBD creams are often applied to the skin to ease muscle or joint pain. Most topicals don't enter the bloodstream. Instead, they affect local cannabinoid receptors in the skin.

Dosage

Talk with a doctor about which CBD brands and products may be best for you and at what dosage you should start your treatment.

When starting any new drug or supplement, it's usually best to start with a low dose. This way you can see how well you tolerate it and whether it's effective at that dose.

Side effects of CBD

An extensive review of CBD's existing clinical data and animal studies reported that CBD is safe and has few, if any, side effects for adults.

Most common side effects are:

• fatigue

• nausea

• changes in appetite

• changes in weight

Interactions

Since CBD is often used in addition to other prescriptions or over-the-counter drugs, more research is needed to understand how the cannabinoid interacts with other meds.

Using CBD may increase or inhibit another drug's effectiveness or side effects. Talking with a doctor or pharmacist can provide you more information about your particular risks.

Why People With Type 2 Diabetes Are Considering CBD

One thing is for sure about CBD: People with type 2 diabetes are taking an interest in the ingredient as a management tool.

In Nevada, where Dr. Brady used to work as a certified diabetes educator, her patients with type 2 diabetes used CBD for nerve pain. She says patients would use CBD in a tincture or in oils that they rubbed on painful areas, including their feet. Patients could buy CBD at medical marijuana dispensaries, which would offer dosing instructions. "They worried about the impact on their blood sugars," says Brady.

Ultimately, though, Brady says that her patients reported that CBD reduced their nerve pain and improved their blood sugar. She adds that those people who used CBD oils for nerve pain also reported sleeping better.

Heather Jackson, the founder and board president of Realm of Caring in Colorado Springs, Colorado, a nonprofit that focuses on cannabis research and education, also senses an interest in CBD within the diabetes community. "In general, especially if they're not well controlled, people are looking at cannabinoid therapy as an alternative, and usually as an adjunct option," says Jackson, adding that callers have questions about CBD for both blood glucose control and neuropathy pain.

Realm of Caring receives an average of 7,000 inquiries about cannabis a month, Jackson says. The organization keeps a registry of these callers, where they live, and their health conditions. Jackson says that people with type 2 diabetes are not a large percentage of the callers, but they currently have 330 people with diabetes in their database.

Jackson says that Realm of Caring does not offer medical advice, and it does not grow or sell cannabis. Instead, it offers education for clients and doctors about cannabis, based on its ever-growing registry of CBD users, their conditions, side effects, and administration regimen. "We are basically educating," says Jackson. "We want you to talk to your doctor about the information you receive."

How Type 2 Diabetes and Anxiety Are Connected

Despite interest among people with type 2 diabetes, large, rigorous studies showing how CBD may affect type 2 diabetes are lacking, says Y. Tony Yang, MPH, a doctor of science in health policy and management and a professor at George Washington University in Washington, DC. Specifically absent are randomized controlled trials, which are the gold standard of medical research, per a June 2016 article in the New England Journal of Medicine.

But early research may suggest the two are worth studying further. For example, a small study published in October 2016 in Diabetes Care in the United Kingdom of 62 people with type 2 diabetes found that CBD did not lower blood glucose. Participants were not on insulin, nor were they on any diabetes drugs, and they were randomly assigned to five different treatment groups for 15 weeks: 100 milligrams (mg) of CBD twice daily; 5 mg of THCV (another chemical in cannabis) twice daily; 5 mg CBD and 5 mg THCV together twice daily; 100 mg CBD and 5 mg of THCV together twice daily; or placebo. According to the authors, THCV (but not CBD) significantly improved blood glucose control.

A Canadian study published in Pain of 37 people with diabetes found that a synthetic cannabinoid called nabilone improved nerve pain. "We also found patients had better sleep measures, so their sleep was more complete. Anxiety levels improved to a smaller amount," says Dr. Toth, who led the study.

"Pain has a lot of neighbors," Toth says. "If you have chronic pain, you typically have sleep issues, raised levels of anxiety, and depression. So, we thought nabilone could target some of those important features in those patients [with diabetic nerve pain]." He adds that nabilone is commonly prescribed for pain in Canada.

Other CBD research is still evolving. Some CBD and diabetes studies have been done in rats, which leads to findings that don't always apply to human health. Other studies have looked more generally at the body's endocannabinoid system, which sends signals about pain, stress, sleep, and other important functions. Still other studies, including one published in the American Journal of Medicine, have looked at marijuana and diabetes, but not CBD specifically.